Foods 7

MW01094337

Complete Guide to Healthy Eating
Includes 30 Day Meal Plan
Recipe's Include:

No Gluten, Dairy, Sugar, or Flour
Vegan & Non-Vegan Options
With Proper Food Combing

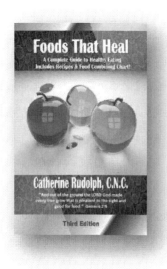

Catherine Rudolph, C.N.C

The information presented herein by Catherine Rudolph is intended for educational purposes only, and to be a supplement to nutrition and health coaching. These statements have not been evaluated by the FDA and are not intended to diagnose, cure, treat or prevent disease. Individual results may vary, and before using any supplements, it is always advisable to consult with your own health care provider.

Table of Contents

Web links available with eBook Version

Introduction

About 13 years ago I lived on a diet consisting of Diet Coke, bread, ice cream, pizza...and no fruits or vegetables. I suffered chronic fatigue, poor digestion, headaches, allergies, and unexplained chronic pain. After about 13 doctors were unable to help me, I decided to take matters into my own hands.

As a result, I found true healing through diet changes, cleansing, fasting, whole food supplementation, and healing prayer. Now as a certified nutrition consultant, the Lord has blessed me with the ability to help others through their own journey to healing.

Dedications

I want to thank my husband, Kurt, for all the years he has stood by me and loved me through my own journey to healing. I would not be where I am today without you Kurt.

I also want to thank Nancy Brush for her ministry to me during some of the most difficult years of my healing, and for showing me the love of Jesus. Your friendship is priceless to me Nancy.

A special thanks to Marie Andorfer and Katherine Brooks for their editing assistance and making this book possible.

Dietary Guidelines For Health:
3 Things Everyone Needs

1. <u>Diet</u>   Eat Foods That Heal

- Clean Water
- Fruits & Vegetables
- *Unrefined* Sea Salt
- Healthy Fats
- Complex Carbs
- Clean Protein

Avoid Foods That Make You Sick

- Tap Water
- Processed Foods
- Refined Salt
- Bad Fats
- Refined Carbs
- Unhealthy Proteins

2. <u>Digestion</u> (and Detox)

You can eat all the right foods and still not feel well if your digestion is compromised, because undigested food will rot in your intestines and becomes a breeding ground for disease (ex. yeast, inflammation, IBS, & more)

- *21 day detox* (refer to my book "Detox Diet")
- Incorporate *proper food combining*
- Nourish & balance gut bacteria
- Take digestive enzymes (& chew your food)

3. <u>Deficiencies</u>

Supplement specific nutritional deficiencies with whole food nutritional supplements.

Statistics & Facts

➢ Research at Oxford University shows that 70% of cancer cases are diet related.

➢ Research also shows that chronic stress, or rather the inability to cope with stress, is responsible for 85-95% of all diseases. *Andreas Mortiz, The Liver and Gallbladder Miracle Cleanse*

➢ According to the International Diabetes Federation, every 10 seconds 2 people develop Diabetes.

How the body regenerates itself into a whole new you

➢ Every 4 days your **stomach lining** replaces itself.

➢ Every 4 weeks the outer layer of our **skin** is replaced

➢ Every 6 weeks you have a **new liver**

➢ Every 2 months almost every cell in our **heart muscle, cartilage, and joints** are rebuilt

➢ Every 2 months you have a **new brain**

➢ Every 3 months you have a **new skeletal structure**

➢ And the **entire human body**, right down to the last atom, is replaced every 5-7 years

ref: Brant Lambert

Disease takes time to develop
A person who smokes might feel fine for years, but cancer is likely developing behind the scenes. By the time you have a symptom, you have been unhealthy for a long time.

Drinks That Heal

"Clean" Water

Our bodies are 70 percent water. We NEED water to live.

Drink half your weight in fluid ounces of purified room temperature water, up to 100 ounces every day, 30 minutes before, or an hour after your meals.

- Hydrates: 85% of headaches are result of dehydration.
- Water prevents fatigue, stress, anxiety, depression
- Boosts Energy & Immune System
- Flushes out toxins that make us sick.
- Promotes weight loss by preventing toxic build up.
- Prevents and eliminates constipation

Best Water Choice:

- **Reverse Osmosis Water** - best choice over all, filters out almost all impurities. (need to re-mineralize)

- **Add PURE mineral drops** to re-mineralize (electrolytes), naturally balance pH (alkalize), optimize weight loss, deliver minerals and oxygen to the cells (creating an environment for health), and flush toxins out at a cellular level.

- **Add Fresh Lemon** for Vitamin C, potassium, wake up & cleanse digestive system, flush toxins, alkalize.

<u>Drinks to Avoid</u>

Poor Water Choices:

- **Tap Water (acidic, full of toxins, void of nutrients)**
  Tap water contains disease causing toxins, pollutants, parasites, bacteria, lead, aluminum, mercury, pesticides, and fluoride & chlorine which have been shown to lead to thyroid disease.
  If your water is acidic, full of toxins, and void of nutrients, it will just run right through you and leave you dehydrated and toxic.
- **Spring Water** - Contains minerals the body cannot use, which can deposit in the blood and joints.
- **Carbon Filtered Tap**
  Removes chlorine, but does not remove fluoride, lead, mercury, nickel, etc.
- **Soft Water**
  Can lead to or exacerbate high blood pressure.

Soft Drinks & Sugar Drinks

Soda, alcohol, Kool-Aide, Juice Boxes, Bottled Juices... All contain sugar, and <u>sugar feeds disease</u> and physically changes and damages our bodies at a cellular level.

Soft drinks are also loaded with artificial food colorings and chemicals which have been shown to cause DNA damage and have been linked to cancer, neurological damage, and many other chronic health conditions.

Two cans of soda can suppress the immune system by 92% for up to 5 hours. Dr. Kenneth Bock

A single can of soda a day can add up to 15 pounds a year.

Coffee:

Contains **Caffeine** which is an agent that temporarily increases body or organ function and increases activity in the central nervous system. Caffeine stresses the organs, especially the adrenal glands, which are designed to handle our *normal* daily stress. Adding stimulants will put your body in high gear, only to crash later, and eventually drain you completely of your energy and health. Stimulants are often addictive as well.

Consider the consequences if you are a coffee drinker:

- Hormonal imbalances as a result of over-stimulating the adrenal glands.
- Dehydration - fluid loss, it interferes with the body's ability to use water.
- Calcium Loss - from acidic blood - leading to osteoporosis because calcium is pulled out of bones to buffer the acids.
- Depletes B vitamins as a result of forcing the body to exert bursts of energy repeatedly.
- Recurring infections - liver has to work hard to process coffee, it is not food and contains chemicals.
- Contribute to Rheumatoid arthritis and stroke
- Raises blood pressure, increased risk of heart attack
- High in pesticides
- Nervousness/Anxiety & Insomnia
- Headaches
- Memory problems
- Food cravings
- Damaged blood vessels
- Raised insulin levels
- Heart palpitations
- Gout & Kidney Stones

> There are studies that have stated coffee has health benefits. However... just like anything else, you have to consider the pro's **and** the con's.

Whole Foods That Heal

Whole Foods
A whole food is any food found in nature in its natural state- not processed in any way. A whole food can be picked off a tree or bush.
Ex) Fresh raw fruits and vegetables, raw whole grains, raw nuts & seeds. Not frozen, canned, or in a box...

Fresh
Unprocessed, not frozen, not canned, not made into flour...bread is not a fresh food. Fresh means found in nature on a tree or bush.

Raw/Living
Raw food is fresh food with enzymes still active. Our diets should ideally be 80% raw food.

Enzymes
String of amino acids forming large protein molecules found in all living things. When you bite into an apple and it turns brown, it is because the LIVE enzymes in the food are starting the digestive process breaking down the apple. Cooking food kills the enzymes in the food.

Fiber
Fiber is the part of food that is not digested. Lowers cholesterol & fat levels in the blood, cleanses intestinal tract.

Ph Balanced Foods (alkaline/acid)
75-80% of our diet needs to be alkaline (the remaining 20-25% needs to be acidic). Our bodies need a healthy balance. Acidosis (when we become too acidic) is very common in our society due to all the processed foods available to us and creates an environment for disease. I do not get hung up on testing my Ph or obsessing over how alkaline or acidic I am, because that in itself can cause stress which will instantly cause the body to be acidic!

Emotions have a huge part to play in the alkalinity and acidity of our bodies. That said, it is still very important to consume a good amount of alkaline foods as a regular part of your diet.

The simplest way to ensure you are getting enough alkaline foods is to focus on consuming plenty of fresh fruits and vegetables. If you do not get the RDA of 9-13 fruits and vegetables in each day, I would highly recommend a good quality green foods powder with fruits, veggies, probiotics, enzymes, and other super foods to fill in the gap.

Again, it's all about balance and being aware without getting too hung up on ph. I also do not recommend trying to alter your ph with high doses of calcium or special waters. That is not natural and your body is smart enough to figure that out. Just remember, balance is what you are aiming for.

Vegetables: Alkalizing

Fruits: Alkalizing with the exception of blueberries, cranberries, and plums, which are more acidifying.

Fruit or Vegetable Juices: Fresh juices are alkalizing. Bottled juices are acidifying.

Proteins: Animal flesh proteins are acidifying, including dairy (due to processing). Plant proteins are alkalizing.

Nuts and Seeds: Primarily alkalizing.

Legumes (beans): Acidifying, but still very healthy.

Sweeteners: Stevia is alkalizing; all sugar and fake sweeteners are extremely acidifying and unhealthy.

Grains: Most are acidifying. However, quinoa, buckwheat, and millet are alkalizing.

Preservatives, Chemicals, & Drugs: Very acidifying and toxic.

Coffee & Soda: Extremely acidifying and very unhealthy.

Herbs & Spices: Alkalizing

Fruits and Vegetables - A perfect whole food

- Reduces risk of disease such as cancer, diabetes, heart disease.
- Lowers blood pressure.
- Cleanses the digestive system.
- Contain antioxidants.
- Prevents obesity.
- Strengthens immune system.
- Contains essential vitamins, minerals, and fiber.

Tips For Eating More Fruits and Veggies:

- Clean & prepare fruits and veggies ahead of time so they are easy to snack on.
- Have a meal of just vegetables.
- Have a vegetable with every meal, and make it the largest portion on your plate..
- Keep fruit where you can see it, you will be more likely to eat it.
- Explore the produce section and try something you have never tried before every time you shop.
- Store in "Green Bags" to keep them fresh longer.
- Juice your veggies
- Make a Green Smoothie

Healthiest Ways to Eat Fruits and Vegetables:

- Fresh is best, frozen is acceptable, avoid canned, as this process depletes the nutrients.
- Vegetables should be eaten raw or gently cooked, can be eaten as snack or with meals.
- Fruit should be eaten for breakfast only with no other food group.

Whole Grains

- Amaranth
- Millet
- Buckwheat
- Rice
- Oats
- Quinoa*

Whole grain bread is **not** a whole grain; there is no bread tree :)

Cheerios are **not** a whole grain food. There is no "Cheerio tree".

White Rice: even white rice is **not** technically a whole grain because the bran and germ have been stripped off and all that is left is the shell, which is only a part of the whole grain.

Whole grain rice flour is **not** a whole grain. It has been highly processed and stripped of most of its nutrients.

*Technically quinoa is a seed, however it properly food combines as a starch.

Raw Nuts & Seeds - Raw, Soaked, Sprouted

Nuts and Seeds should always be eaten raw after soaking in water for 10-12 hours (and set out to dry if desired)

Why Soak Nuts & Seeds?

- **Increase Digestibility:** By neutralizing enzyme inhibitors (a naturally occurring nut preservative).

- **Eliminate Phytic Acid:** That inhibits the absorption of vital minerals.

- **Increase Nutrient Absorption:** (vitamins, minerals, proteins & phytonutrients).

Nuts and seeds naturally contain enzyme inhibitors so they can wait until weather conditions are right for growth before they germinate. These enzyme inhibitors act as a preservative for the nut, making sure it can stay viable for a long time.

As spring rain comes, nuts & seeds sit in the water and slowly begin to lose this inhibitor, allowing for germination to take place.

However, farmers pick the nuts & seeds, dry them, and ship them to your grocer to be put on a shelf for sale while this enzyme inhibitor is still intact.

This is why nuts have a reputation as being difficult to digest. The inhibitor actually inhibits digestion when nuts are eaten without undergoing the process nature intended.

Not only that, but un-soaked nuts actually neutralize the enzymes your body uses to control inflammation and aid digestion. Eating un-soaked nuts is extremely hard on the digestive system and calls for the pancreas to produce huge amounts of digestive enzymes to counteract the inhibitor.

Note: Sprouting nuts and seeds is another step you can take to make them even more digestible.

Do I always have to buy organic?

Ideally organic is always the best choice. However, it can be difficult to find organic, and it can get very expensive!

I always buy organic meat to avoid the antibiotics and growth hormones injected in non-organically raised animals. We are eating whatever the animal eats.

Roughly 70 percent of total US antibiotic production -- are fed to chickens, pigs, and cows for non-therapeutic purposes like growth promotion, according to a new report from the Union of Concerned Scientists.

As far as fresh fruits and vegetables are concerned, it is helpful to have a list of which fruits and vegetables are sprayed the least with pesticides and which are sprayed the most.

The following list is put out by the environmental Working Group ranking highest and lowest sprayed produce. When you can't always buy organic, this is a great list to help you prioritize buying organic versus non-organic.

Dirty Dozen: Highest in Pesticides (best to buy organic)

1. Celery
2. Peaches
3. Strawberries
4. Apples
5. Blueberries
6. Nectarines
7. Bell Peppers
8. Spinach
9. Cherries
10. Kale/Collard greens
11. White Potatoes
12. Imported grapes

Healthy 15: Lowest in Pesticides

1. Onions
2. Avocados
3. Sweet Corn
4. Pineapple
5. Mangos
6. Sweet Peas
7. Asparagus
8. Kiwi
9. Cabbage
10. Eggplant
11. Cantaloupe
12. Watermelon
13. Grapefruit
14. Sweet Potato
15. Honeydew Melon

Avoid Processed Foods

*Processed food is any food that is altered from its whole food state, often containing **preservatives** added to lengthen shelf life.*

- Tell-tale sign you are looking at processed food? Uniform appearance, long shelf-life, instant results, in wrapper or can, contain artificial flavors, read label...

- Processed foods not only don't provide any nutrients, but actually rob our bodies of essential nutrients.

- **Examples** of processed foods: bread, dry cereal, deserts, roasted nuts, popcorn, rice meals, chips, frozen meals, deli meat, salad dressings...basically any food in a bag, can, bottle or box is very likely to be processed. Read the label carefully, the longer the ingredient list, the worse it is.

Avoid Preservatives

Preservatives are chemical compounds that are added to protect against decay and decomposition. I will list a few, but there is no way I could list them all because there are thousands of them. So the best rule to follow is:

If you can't read it, don't eat it.

- **MSG:** some known side effects of this preservative

Seizures	Headaches
Brain cell death	Strokes
Brain damage	Hypoglycemia
Allergies	Brain Tumors

Russell Blaylock "Excitotoxins the Taste that Kills"

- **Sulfates & sulfites**
- **nitrates & nitrites**
- **BHT**
- **Natural flavors**
- **Food coloring**

A few common side effects of Preservatives:

Make you crave sugar.

Cause weight problems, empty calories, cause food cravings.

Block nutrients from being absorbed.

Overworks and congests the liver as it tries to process and detoxify the body from these foreign chemicals

Carcinogenic

Salt that Heals

Unrefined Sea Salt ~ is vital for good health

- Helps to regulate the water content in your body. Without it, you will dehydrate over time showing classic symptoms like asthma, arthritis, high blood pressure, edema, allergies, etc.

- Is effective in stabilizing irregular heartbeats and, contrary to the misconception that it causes high blood pressure, it is essential for the regulation of blood pressure - in conjunction with water. Naturally the proportions are critical.

- Vital to the extraction of excess acidity from the cells in the body, particularly the brain cells.

- Vital for balancing the sugar levels in the blood

- Vital to the nerve cells' communication and information processing all the time that the brain cells work, from the moment of conception to death.

- Vital for absorption of food particles through the intestinal tract.

- Vital for the clearance from the lungs of mucus plugs and sticky phlegm, particularly in asthma and cystic fibrosis.

- Salt is vital for clearing up catarrh and sinus congestion.

- Strong natural antihistamine.

- Essential for the prevention of muscle cramps.

- Vital to prevent excess saliva production to the point that it flows out of the mouth during sleep. Needing to constantly mop up excess saliva indicates salt shortage

- Vital to making the structure of bones firm. Osteoporosis is a result of salt and water shortage in the body.

- Vital for sleep regulation.

- Vital for the prevention of gout and gouty arthritis.

- Vital for maintaining libido.

- Vital for preventing varicose veins and spider veins.

Ref: Miracle Salt by Mae M. Vander Boom
Ref: Liver and Gallbladder by Andrea Moritz

Salt to Avoid

Refined Salt

Salt that is stripped of all its minerals (besides sodium and chloride) and heated at such high temperatures that the chemical structure of the salt changes. It is chemically cleaned and bleached and treated with anti-caking agents, so it does not dissolve and combine with the water and fluids present in our bodies as is needed.

Things to be aware of:

- Bouillon is not sea salt therefore not a healthy option.
- Almost all restaurant food contains liberal amounts of refined salt.
- Most processed foods contain refined salt.
- Labels can read "sea salt" and still be refined and unhealthy.

Side Effects Include

Salt build up in the body leaving deposits in organs and tissue, causing severe health problems, can lead to edema, high blood pressure, exercise induced asthma, heartburn and osteoporosis. Refined salt is in most processed foods.

Carbohydrates That Heal

Complex Carbohydrates

Carbohydrates have gotten a bad rap in the past few years. But not all carbs are equal. Vegetables are "carbs", and they are one of the most nutrient dense foods on the planet because they are "complex" carbohydrates. Complex carbohydrates are derived from plants - vegetables, whole grains, beans, nuts & seeds, and they are the body's main source of energy. Complex carbohydrates:

- Contain complete nutrients

- High in fiber

- Improve digestion

- Provide energy

- Digest more slowly which helps balance blood sugar

Buckwheat	Brussels Sprouts
Brown Rice	Cabbage
Quinoa	Carrots
Wheat Germ	Cauliflower
Spelt	Celery
Artichoke	Collard Greens
Arugula	Cucumber
Asparagus	Endive
Bok Choy	Fennel
Broccoli	Garlic

Jicama	Radishes
Kale	Rutabaga
Leeks	Scallions
Lettuce (Romaine)	Squash
Mustard greens	Spinach
Okra	Sprouts
Onions	Swiss Chard
Nappa	Tomato
Parsley	Turnips
Peppers	Sweet Potato

Note: Whole Grain -Hull (used in bread for longer shelf life - no nutrients), Bran (some nutrients), Germs (most nutrients)

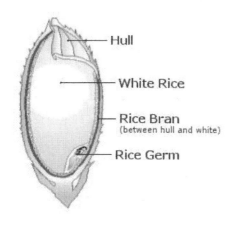

Carbohydrates to Avoid

Refined Processed Carbohydrates

Refined Carbohydrates are grains that have been overly processed to improve shelf life.

Nutrient Deficient

Most of the vitamins and minerals are removed in the processing, which leaves the food to act as pure sugar when you eat it. And the vitamins that are "added" are unusable by our bodies, i.e. "enriched".

Side Effects of Refined Carbohydrates

- Sugar cravings
- Mood swing
- Irritability
- Blood sugar imbalances
- Weight gain
- Malnutrition
- Constipation
- Congestion
- Disease

Examples of Refined Carbohydrates

- White rice
- White potatoes
- Dry (cold) cereals
- White bread
- Most snack foods
- Chips
- Cookies
- Sweets
- Cakes
- Bagels

Wheat and Gluten:

Wheat contains gluten which makes it difficult to digest whether you have sensitivity to it or not. And unfortunately, gluten is added to so many of our foods, we become sensitive as a result of consuming it way too much by default. Gluten is what makes bread so fluffy.

Mucus Producing:

The gluten in wheat creates a mucous in the body, the same kind of mucous that you get when you have a sinus cold. And if there is mucous stored up in our bodies, it gives bad bacteria a nice secure hiding place to create further problems.

Inflammatory Agent:

Gluten is a hard to digest protein that can also contribute to Candida, arthritis, sinusitis, constipation, IBS, celiac, liver & gall bladder congestion, insomnia, suppressed immune system, and depression.

Gluten Grains:

- Barley
- Kamut
- Oats
- Rye
- Teft
- Wheat

Non-Gluten Grains:

- Amaranth
- Quinoa
- Rice
- Millet
- Buckwheat

Fats

Why Do We Need Fat?

- Our brains are 70% fat, we need to feed our brains!
- Vitamins A, D, E and K are all fat soluble, the body cannot use these vitamins without healthy fats
- Fat slows down digestion which helps suppress appetite
- Helps reduce food cravings
- Necessary for healthy hormonal balance
- Necessary for healthy skin
- Prevent stagnant bile which leads to gallbladder stones

Fats That Heal

Essential Fatty Acid's

Omega 3's and Omega 6's - both essential to the body, cannot be made by the body, need to come from dietary sources. Omega 3 is often deficient in our diets.

Why you need Omega 3's

- Lower cholesterol, triglyceride levels, & blood pressure
- Excellent "brain food" as it helps with mental clarity, focus, and can be especially beneficial for those with ADD & ADHD
- Reduce anxiety
- Stabilize blood sugar

- Reduce the risk of breast, prostate, and colon cancers

- Improve digestion

- Help with weight loss

- Basic anti-inflammatory that can relieve pain and tissue damage caused by rheumatoid arthritis, osteoporosis, lupus, osteoporosis, irritable colon, diverticulitis, gastritis, enteritis, breast cancer, chronic constipation.

Foods High In Omega 3

- **Flaxseeds:** are great for the essential fatty acids, but they are also a great source of fiber. You can buy the whole seed, and then grind them daily in a coffee grinder. The oil is very susceptible to rancidity. So if you buy the oil, store it in a dark bottle in the refrigerator or freezer. Never heat flaxseed oil.

- **Chia Seeds:** are another great source of essential fatty acids, and you do not need to grind the seed. They are also high in Vitamins A, B, E, and D, and minerals including calcium, phosphorus, potassium, sulfur, iron, iodine, copper, zinc, sodium, magnesium, manganese, niacin, thiamine, silicon, and anti-oxidants.

- **Fish Oil:** I avoid fish oil due to over processing.

- **Kale:** not only is kale high in omega 3's, it is also an alkaline food, loaded with nutrients, a cancer fighter, high in calcium, magnesium, iron, and contains twice as much protein as steak (per every 100 calories).

- **Walnuts:** Most nuts are higher in omega 6's, which can create an omega 3 deficiency. Walnuts are the one nut that is actually higher in omega 3's. Make sure you buy them raw and soak them for 12 hours before you eat them.

Omega 3 Deficiencies can lead to:

- Depression
- Weight gain
- Allergies
- Eczema
- Inflammation
- Weak Immune System
- Cancer
- Arthritis
- Diabetes
- ADD/ADHD
- Fatigue
- Dry Skin
- Dandruff
- Heart Disease
- Hyperactivity
- Irritability

Other Healthy Fats

Olive Oil

Olive oil contains oleic acid which aids in keeping our arteries supple and helps prevent cancer. It is also high in antioxidants, including Vita E, and has been shown to be effective in colon cancer prevention.

*Do not cook with olive oil; high heat damages this oil and will lead to free radicals. Free radicals are responsible for aging and tissue damage. They can even lead to cancer.

Coconut Oil

Great for cooking, handles high heat well. In addition, it helps:

- Increase metabolism for weight Loss

- Prevent Heart Diseases

- Healing for Pancreatitis

- Healing to Digestion

- Boost Immune System

- Fight Infection

- Detoxify Liver

- Prevent Diabetes

Ghee (Clarified Butter)

Ghee is clarified butter, meaning the milk solids, proteins, water, and impurities are removed.

- Can handle high heat for cooking and baking without being damaged

- Aids Digestion

- Helps body assimilate nutrients

- It is said to be anti-cancer, anti-viral

- Non Dairy

Fats To Avoid

Trans Fats

Trans Fats are the result of an artificial process of converting oil into a more stable/solid form, like margarine. This process is called hydrogenation.

The purpose of Trans Fats is to allow a longer shelf life. But trans fats are one of the worst things you can put in your body. Even 1/2 gram per day can quickly take your health in the wrong direction.

Consuming trans-fats can increase your risk of:

- High cholesterol
- Type II diabetes
- Liver dysfunction
- Breast cancer
- Prostate cancer

Below are a few examples of foods that contain Trans Fats:

- **French Fries:** (a medium order) contain 14.5 grams.
- **Donuts:** contain about 5 grams of trans fats each.
- **Spreads:** Margarine and shortening.
- **Baked Goods:** Cookies and cakes.
- **Ramen Noodles:** are very high in trans fats!

Heated/Refined Fats

The **only** fats that are safe to cook with are ghee and coconut oil. High heat will damage all other fats, leading to free radicals. Free radicals are responsible for aging and tissue damage. They can even lead to cancer. Ex) All potato chips, because they have been fried at high heat, all baked goods with oil on the list, all crackers, cookies..

I highly recommend you avoid all vegetable oils, ESPECIALLY Canola oil, which is in EVERY thing.

Protein

Guidelines and Facts

- Buy Organic Meat. According to a government study, over 90% of the chickens in this country are infected with leukosis (chicken cancer). *Ref: John Barron Lessons from the Miracle Doctors.*

- Red Meat? According to a study at Harvard Medical School, "Men who eat red meat as a main dish five or more times a week have 4 times the risk of colon cancer than men who eat red meat less than once a month...they are also twice as likely to get prostate cancer" .

- Choose lean meats and limit meats high in saturated fats.

- Eat a variety to ensure you get all 22 amino acids.

- Heavy consumption of meat compromises beneficial bacteria in the colon, increasing the levels of harmful bacteria in the colon.

- High consumption of meat also tends to increase over-all acidity in the body, which can increase the risk of other health problems including higher risk of osteoporosis and cancer.

- Is a vegetarian diet better? Can be better for colon health but can create vitamin/mineral deficiencies.

- Video "The Truth About Eating Meat- Dr Michael Klaper"

Proteins That Heal

- Chicken (organic)
- Hemp Seeds, Chia Seeds
- Turkey (organic)
- Fish (wild caught)
- Eggs
- Sprouted Nuts & Seeds
- Quinoa & Buckwheat
- Hemp Seeds or Chia Seeds
- Nutritional Yeast
- Bee Pollen
- Spirulina or Chlorella
- Goat Milk, Goat Yogurt, Goat Cheese
- Lima Beans, Green Peas

Definitions Related to Protein

Enzymes - strings of amino acids forming large protein molecules found in all living things.

Amino Acids- building blocks of protein.

Proteins - Sequence of amino acids and all raw foods contain protein because all raw food contains live enzymes.

<u>Proteins to Avoid</u>

- Cow Milk, Cheese, yogurt

- Unfermented Soy & Tofu

- Whey (protein shakes)

- Anything Fried

- Beef, Pork (bacon, sausage, ham)

- Deli Meat, Hot Dogs

- Meat with growth hormones or antibiotics

- Peanuts are also not a good option for the following reasons:

  1. Peanuts tend to grow mold quickly.
  2. Peanuts block iodine absorption.

Dairy That Heals

Goats Milk

Raw Milk from grass-fed, pastured cattle can actually improve health in the areas of allergies, chronic fatigue, immune system, digestion, infection, & autism. Also contains enzymes, essential EFAs, vitamins, minerals, and beneficial bacteria.

A few non-dairy options for calcium are almonds (93mg), broccoli (178mg), chia seeds (177mg). *(milk contains 300mg/cup)*

Dairy To Avoid

Don't we need to eat dairy to get our calcium? "Milk does the body good," right? But does milk really do the body good? Is it as healthy as it is presented on television commercials? After all, milk is mentioned in the Bible. Abraham gave milk to the visiting angels in Genesis 18:18. And God described the promise land in Exodus 3:8 as flowing with milk and honey. So if God created it, it must be good. Right? It depends on whether it is consumed in its natural raw form, or in a commercially denatured, toxic form.

Pasteurized, Homogenized Milk

Now ranks as the number one food allergy in the US. Kurt Oster, MD, Chief of Cardiology and Chairman of the Department of Medicine at Park City Hospital in Bridgeport, CT states "Milk has been changed over the years by processing into an unrecognizable physiochemical emulsion which bears very little resemblance to the original, natural, and nutritional milk."

- **Difficult to Digest**
  How many times have we heard "I am dairy intolerant". Processed dairy is difficult to digest, it is also another common allergen, it creates gastrointestinal distress, gas, bloating, constipation, diarrhea, acid reflux, & liver/gallbladder congestion.

- **Mucous Producing**
  Clogs the tissues and organs resulting in congestion and inflammation, which again leads to disease.

- **Strong Inflammatory**
  Again, due to the mucus producing nature of dairy that clogs vital organs.

- **Exacerbates & Causes respiratory problems**
  Asthma
  Sinus infections
  Allergies

- **Cancer Causing (Carcinogen)**
  As a result of added growth hormones

- **Contains Antibiotics**
  Which leads antibiotic resistance & bowel disease

- **Highly Processed - Homogenization and Pasteurization**
  Destroys enzymes, proteins, vitamins, minerals, & beneficial bacteria. Results in loss of up to 60% of its fat-soluble vitamins, and up to 50% loss of Vitamin C. Vitamins B6 and B12 are completely destroyed, and 38%-80% of the water-soluble vitamins are destroyed. Synthetic D is often added back into commercial milk, further unbalancing the nutrient profile. The synthetic form of Vitamin D promotes calcification of soft tissues and softening of hard tissue such as bones. Calcium availability is decreased by 50% or more as well.

Diseases Associated with Pasteurized, Homogenized Milk are:

- Excess Mucous
- Allergies
- Anemia
- Skin Rashes
- Osteoporosis
- Type 2 Diabetes
- Digestive Problems
- Heart Disease
- Kidney Disease
- MS
- Cancer
- Recurrent ear Infections
- Behavioral Problems
- Autism
- Mood Swings
- Depression

What are some common dairy foods?

Milk, yogurt, cottage cheese, cheese, butter, creamy salad dressings, creamer, casein, whey

Video / Research Web Links (with eBook version)

Video "The Truth About Dairy – Dr. Gregor

Video "Dairy Asthma and RA – Dr. Gregor

Prostate Cancer and Dairy

Acne and Dairy

Pus in Cheese

Parkinson's and Dairy

Lung, Breast, & Ovarian Cancer and Dairy

Colon Cancer and Dairy

Feces and Raw Milk

Soy That Heals

If you want to add soy to your diet, fermented forms are the only form that can be digested by your body. These include:

- Tempeh
- Tamari
- Natto
- Miso

Soy To Avoid

(Avoid any soy that is not fermented)

- Soy phytoestrogens are potent anti-thyroid agents that cause hypothyroid and may cause thyroid cancer

- Soy contains trypsin inhibitors that interfere with protein digestion and may cause pancreatic disorders

- Soy phytoestrogens disrupt endocrine function and have the potential to cause infertility and can promote breast cancer

- Soy foods increase the bodies requirement for vitamin D

- MSG, a potent neurotoxin, is formed during soy food processing

- Soy foods contain high levels of aluminum which is toxic to the nervous system and kidneys

  Ref: The Weston A. Price Foundation

Sweeteners That Heal

Sweeteners that heal include: (in moderation)

- <u>Raw</u> Honey
- Stevia

Sweeteners To Avoid

Sugar

When you eat sugar, your liver turns it into fat, which in turn spills into the blood, raising LDL levels in the blood, clogging the arteries.

Sugar can also cause:

- Increased risk of diabetes by 85%
- Weaker immune system
- Inflammation
- Headaches
- Exacerbated PMS & hormonal imbalances
- Asthma
- Arthritis
- Gallstones
- Kidney stones
- Osteoporosis
- Candida (yeast overgrowth)
- Depression
- Food allergies

- Increases risk of Cardiovascular disease
- Hyperactivity
- Weight gain
- Sugar is addictive. It activates the same part of the brain as cocaine

Names for Sugar

- corn syrup
- fructose
- dextrose
- glucose
- maltodextrine
- maltose
- erythritol

- galactose
- high fructose
- corn syrup
- rice syrup
- sucrose
- agave (not healthy)

Artificial Sweeteners

Artificial sweeteners are chemicals used to replace sugar, aka poison and very dangerous in the body.

Common Names for fake sweeteners:

Sucralose, splenda, aspartame, sweet and low, equal...

Foods that fake sweeteners are found in:

Protein bars, whey protein shakes, yogurts, diet sodas, teas, gums...

Side Effects of Aspartame

- Migraines

- Seizures

- Tumors

- Dizziness/Vertigo

- Blurred vision

- Gastrointestinal problems

- Allergic reactions

- Rise in Blood sugar

- Weight gain

- Fertility problems

- Gout

- Hypothyroidism

- Neurological disorders

- Fluid retention

- Yeast Overgrowth

- Sugar cravings

- Swelling of the kidneys

- Weakened immune system

- Increase of infections due to up to 50 % reduction of friendly bacteria in intestines

There is nothing "better" about using an artificial sweetener in place of sugar. The pancreas will still overproduce insulin. There are many other options that will protect your body from the inevitable disease that will manifest as a result of these fake foods that are not food at all.

Digestion

What is digestion?

It is the process by which food is converted into substances that can be absorbed and assimilated by the body.

When we eat our food, it needs to be broken down enough to enter into and nourish our cells. If our digestion is weak, our food will not be broken down enough. Food will ferment in the intestinal tract and turn into waste. This is a huge problem because parasites and Candida (a yeast like fungus) feed on undigested food, multiply like crazy, and make us sick. Undigested food is the root problem to many diseases. Even with a perfect diet, we cannot be healthy and feel our best if our digestion is not functioning properly.

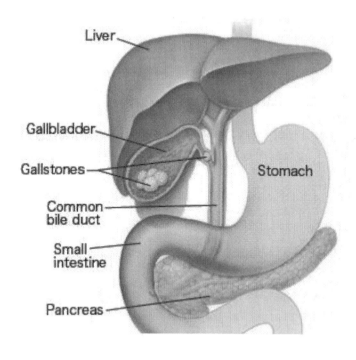

The Digestive Process

1. Mouth

Chewing food is often overlooked in the digestive process. Amylase, Protease, and Lipase are enzymes in the saliva that begin the process of breaking down the food. Some enzymes needed to break down foods do not exist in the body, but they do exist in the food. If you chew your food properly these enzymes will be activated. One of these is cellulase, which is not made by the human body. Vegetables that contain cellulase are covered with a thin coating of cellulose (fiber that aids in smooth working of the intestinal tract). The cellulose must be chewed off because human enzymes cannot penetrate this protective layer. If it is not removed you can develop gas and not get the nutrients from your food. 40-80% of ingested complex carbohydrates can be digested in 15 minutes if chewed properly.

2. Stomach (where proper food combining is important)

When food enters the stomach and begins to stretch the stomach, this signals the body to begin producing hydrochloric acid. It takes about 45 minutes for the acid to be formed. Hydrochloric acid does not digest food, it activates your protein-digestive enzymes, and kills much of the bacteria in your food. Many people have low stomach acid.

Causes of Acid reflux/Heartburn

- Improper food combining - combining food groups that don't digest well together. In this book, every recipe includes proper food combining to maximize digestion.
- Low HCL levels in the stomach cause food to sit in the stomach too long and ferment.
- Back-flushing of toxins, waste, and bile from the intestines into the stomach.
- Reduced mucus production by the stomach as a result of liver congestion and/or gallbladder stones.

- Overeating
- Culprits: Fried foods, coffee, iced drinks, alcohol, dehydration, stress, too much animal protein

3. Duodenum (The top of the small intestines where I like to say all the magic happens :)

At this point the partially digested food is liquid *chyme*. The **pancreas** produces digestive enzymes that act in the duodenum. These enzymes play a major role in digestion. The **liver** produces bile (which is alkaline), sends it to the **gallbladder** where is it stored, then when food is eaten the bile is released into the duodenum (small intestines). Fats are not water-soluble and must be emulsified with bile, which functions as a degreaser. (Bile does not contain enzymes). If bile is not released properly, fat/oils cannot be degreased, and food will not be digested because the enzymes cannot get through the fats.

Symptoms of low Bile Flow: Floating feces, tan or gray feces, shiny feces, foul smelling feces.

4. Small Intestines

The small intestines are where most of the nutrient absorption takes place if all prior phases have properly taken place. Digestive enzymes and probiotics play a critical role in nutrient absorption in the small intestines.

5. Large Intestines/Colon

The colon is the last part of the digestive system. It extracts water and salt from solid wastes before they are eliminated from the body, and is the site in which flora-aided (largely bacteria) fermentation of unabsorbed material occurs. Unlike the small intestine, the colon does not play a major role in absorption of foods and nutrients. However, the colon does absorb water, potassium and some fat-soluble vitamins.

Cleansing the Colon

There is a common phrase you might have heard before "death begins in the colon". How true this is! Whatever food we eat that is not utilized in the body, becomes waste. Most of this waste leaves the body on a daily basis through the colon. However, a huge percentage of the population does not eliminate this waste on a regular basis (at least once daily). When this happens, the poisons back up into the body, and make us tired and unhealthy. Your body will re-absorb theses poisons each day you do not eliminate them and make you sick. Cleansing the colon can improve your health, energy, digestion, and overall well-being.

Note: (colon cleansing is more than a bottle of pills you buy at a health food store or on-line).

The average American stores from 10 to 12 pounds of fecal waste in their colon, which is definitely not healthy. Dr. Schultz

Colon Disease

In 1950, the Merck Manual (the leading medical text on the diagnosis of disease) stated that only 10% of Americans developed bowel disease. Today, it states that 100% of Americans will eventually develop bowel disease (diverticulosis), if they live long enough. Diverticuli (sac-like herniations inside your colon due to excess fecal matter build-up) are a leading precursor to colon cancer. Ref: Dr. Schultz

Bristol Stool Chart

The Bristol Chart was first published in the Scandinavian Journal of Gastroenterology in 1997.

The Ideal bowel movement should occur 2-3 times a day, and be approximately 4-8 inches long, be in one piece, and leave the body with no straining or discomfort. There should be no gas or odor.

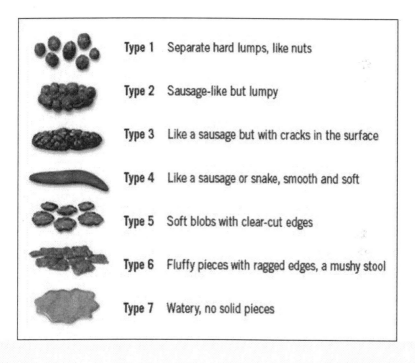

Type 1   Separate hard lumps, like nuts

Type 2   Sausage-like but lumpy

Type 3   Like a sausage but with cracks in the surface

Type 4   Like a sausage or snake, smooth and soft

Type 5   Soft blobs with clear-cut edges

Type 6   Fluffy pieces with ragged edges, a mushy stool

Type 7   Watery, no solid pieces

Type 1: Separate hard lumps, like nuts

Constipation: even if you have daily bowel movements
Possible causes: not enough water, bacterial imbalance, worries, not enough fiber, too much dry food

Type 2: Sausage-like but lumpy

Constipation: To attain this form, the stools must be in the colon for at least several weeks
Possible causes: same as Type 1

Type 3: Like a sausage but with cracks in the surface

Acceptable

Type 4: Like a sausage or snake, smooth and soft

Ideal, easy to pass, this is your goal for optimal health

Type 5: Soft blobs with clear-cut edges

Possible risk of bowel disease and/or bowel toxicity, and need intestinal cleansing

Type 6: Fluffy pieces with ragged edges, a mushy stool
Form of diarrhea
You may be toxic and need intestinal cleansing

Type 7: Watery, no solid pieces

Diarrhea
Probably Causes: lactose intolerance, food poisoning, antibiotics, travel, anxiety, stress, inflammatory bowel disease.

Ref: Living Balanced by Stacey Kimbrell

What Causes Poor Digestion?

- Enzyme Deficiency from cooked food
- Not Chewing Food thoroughly
- Poor Food Choices
- Overeating
- Sugar & Unhealthy fats
- Chemicals & Preservatives
- Low stomach acid
- Antacids – shut down acid production for 9 days
- Liver Congestion
- Chronic Illness
- Chewing gum – changes stomach ph
- Lack of Good Bacteria in the bowel
- Candida overgrowth
- Accumulation of toxins in the body
- Medications
- Stress, Trauma, Surgery

Are you digesting the food you eat?

☐ Eat cooked food

☐ Acid reflux, heart burn, use antacids, ulcers

☐ Bloating after meals (food sits in stomach)

☐ Constipation (less than two full BM/day)

☐ Indigestion, burping, or lower bowel gas

☐ Yeast overgrowth or parasites

☐ Food allergies/intolerances: gluten, dairy...

☐ Food cravings, never satisfied

☐ High meat, carb/sugar, fat diet (circle one)

☐ Liver/gallbladder stones congestion

☐ High cholesterol or blood pressure

☐ Fatigue

☐ Chronic disease: diabetes, heart disease, auto-immune, inflammation, fibromyalgia.

☐ Can't lose weight

☐ Skin conditions (eczema, acne, rosacea...)

If you checked off any of the above symptoms, you are likely in need of a digestive enzyme

10 Ways To Maximize Your Digestion:

1. **Diet**
   Eat *Foods That Heal* and avoid foods that make you sick.

2. **Digestive Enzymes** (and chew your food)
   - Ensures nutrients are easily assimilated by the body because our bodies need food at a cellular level
   - Reduces the digestive burden of the body
   - Prevents toxic bowel from undigested food. Undigested food will ferment and feed yeast & parasites. Bloating and gas occurs, digestion and immune function become weak and now you have toxic bowel.

3. **Probiotics**
   SBO probiotics and cultured foods
   - Stronger immune system
   - Improved digestion alleviating many digestive disorders such as constipation, diarrhea, and IBS
   - Healthier skin even improving eczema & psoriasis, because healthy gut inside = healthy skin outside
   - Replaces healthy bacteria destroyed by antibiotics
   - Increases ability to synthesize vitamin B
   - Increases ability to absorb calcium
   - Promotes anti-tumor & anti-cancer activity in the body
   - Remedy for bad breath

4. **Slow down and chew** your food until it's the consistency of paste.

5. **Drink water** between meals not with meals

6. **Avoid overeating,** it weakens digestion and stresses the organs in your body.

7. **Eat your heaviest meal at lunch** time when digestion is strongest.

8. **Do not eat after 7pm.**

9. **Proper food combining** (view chart page 106)
   - Eat Fruit by itself 2 hours before other food.
   - Never eat proteins with grains/starches
   - Vegetables combine well with anything except fruit
   - Grains/Starches combine well with Oils/Fats.
   - Animal proteins should only be combined with vegetables. Some people also do fine adding fats to flesh proteins, especially if you take digestive enzymes with your meal

10. **Detox** at least three times a year (refer to my book *"Detox Diet" to cleanse colon, kidney, liver, lung, lymph, skin)*

Testing For Food Allergens/Intolerances

The simplest way to figure out what the offending food or foods might be is to do a food elimination diet. My 21-day detox diet is the simplest way to eliminate the most common food allergens.

Refer to my book *"Detox Diet"* to cleanse colon, kidney, liver, lung, lymph & skin.

*If you eat the same food repeatedly day after day, crave certain foods/need them daily for energy, or have any of the following symptoms, you might have a food allergy or sensitivity.

- Acne
- Anxiety
- Arthritis
- Asthma
- ADD
- Bronchitis
- Candida (yeast)
- Chronic Fatigue
- Chron's disease
- Celiac disease
- Diarrhea
- Diabetes
- Depression

- Ear infections
- Gallbladder stones
- Hay fever
- Migraines or headaches
- Hyperactivity
- IBS
- PMS
- Sinusitis
- Skin disorders
- Sleep disorders
- Tonsilitis

Ref: Kelly Hayford's " If It's Not Food Don't Eat It

Most Common Food Allergens

Alcohol	Eggs	Sugars
Fake sweeteners	Tomatoes	Shellfish
Chocolate & cola	Potatoes	Soy
Oranges	Peanuts	Strawberries
Coffee & caffeine	Preservatives	Wheat & gluten
Dairy products	Colorings	Yeast

If you have an actual allergy to a food, as opposed to intolerance, you will have an immediate reaction, i.e. tongue swelling. You need to completely eliminate these foods from your diet, and this type of reaction requires immediate medical attention.

<u>Candida</u> (Yeast Overgrowth)

Candida is a fungus (form of yeast) that naturally occurs in the intestinal tract, mouth, throat, and genitals. In proper balance it performs necessary functions. However, when overgrowth occurs and upsets the healthy balance of bacteria, it becomes a health problem.

I came up with the following analogy to help my clients better understand candida and the delicate balance of bacteria in their gut:

- Grass represents "good bacteria" in your body.
- Weeds represent "bad" strands of candida such as candida albicans.
- Fertilizer represents probiotics (healthy bacteria)
- Weed killer represents antibiotics

Imagine you have a beautiful front yard of green grass. How do you keep it healthy? Fertilizer and water.

In a perfect scenario, if your grass is thick and healthy, weeds will not take over your yard, and you will not need to use weed killer.

Now let's say weeds do start to invade your yard, because the grass is not thick enough to choke them out. What do you do? Kill them with weed killer so they don't get out of control. But if you aren't careful you can kill everything, the weeds AND the grass. And you need grass to choke out future weeds.

Once the weeds have taken over, it becomes this constant battle of trying to grow the grass, while killing the weeds! And it can be a very difficult and frustrating battle.

A similar process happens in your body when you take antibiotics. You kill everything, even the healthy bacteria. Sometimes antibiotics are necessary. However, when you take antibiotics to kill infectious bacteria, you also kill the good guys. And you NEED the good guys. They are a huge part of your immune system. 60% of your immune system resides in your intestines. Healthy bacteria keep candida in proper balance and under control. When you kill the healthy bacteria, bad candida can take over. You end up in this constant battle of trying to replenish your army of good guys, while constantly fighting off the bad guys!

A diet full of sugar and processed food will kill off good bacteria, and feed bad candida. Undigested food will also feed bad candida.

The following is a list of common health conditions that can occur as a result of Candida overgrowth:

- Dramatically reduced immune system

- Conditions, syndromes, and illnesses.

- Accumulation of 70 different toxins into the body

- Digestive health problems

- Nervous system problems

- Cardiovascular health problems

- Endocrine system problems

- Lymphatic congestion

- Musculoskeletal pain

- Candida can burrow holes in the intestinal tract, enter the blood stream, and make its way into other organs in the body

Most Common Causes of Candida/Yeast Overgrowth

- Antibiotics
- Undigested food
- Diet low in healthy fats
- Diet high in sugar, bad fats, and processed food

Test for Candida (Yeast Overgrowth)

Answer "yes" or "no" for the following questions.

1. Do you experience regular fatigue and/or muscle aches and pains?
2. Do you have food sensitivities or food allergies?
3. Have you experienced nail fungus, athlete's foot or jock itch?
4. Do you have any skin disorders?
5. Do you have recurrent vaginal yeast infections?
6. Have you taken broad spectrum antibiotics-even for one period?
7. Do you crave sugar or alcohol?
8. Do you commonly have gas and bloating?
9. Do you suffer from depression or anxiety?
10. Do you crave bread, pasta, or other refined flour?
11. Have you taken birth control pills?
12. Do you experience brain fog?

Answering yes to 3 or more of the above questions indicates you may be suffering from Candida.

The Candida Diet

There are several versions of the candida diet out there, and hundreds, probably thousands of books on the candida diet. But very few of them focus on the root problem, which is poor digestion. The natural sugars in fruit are not the problem. We need glucose for energy. The brain relies on glucose as its main fuel. The inability to digest those natural sugars in fruit is the problem. So when I am working with a client who has yeast overgrowth, I do not focus on killing the bad guys, which is the most common method of dealing with candida. I focus on digestion and enzyme therapy so the digestive system can heal and function properly. Candida feeds on undigested food. If we digest our food properly, candida will not survive.

That said, diet is still very important because soda and refined carbohydrates are not real food. Candida will feed off of undigested food and fake food as well. So instead of putting my clients on some rigid candida diet, I suggest the following protocol:

Candida Diet Guidelines

1. Eat Foods That Heal & Avoid: food allergens, sugar, bad fats, processed foods.

2. Restore Digestion: including digestive enzymes and probiotics. Refer to digestion guidelines on page 48.

3. Cleanse & Detox: keep bile moving and colon clean.

4. Targeted Therapy: Heal the gut lining, consider food based anti-fungals.

10 Tips For Healthy Weight Loss

1. Lifestyle/Default Diet: Eat foods that heal as a lifestyle and avoid processed foods as much as possible. Processed foods contain toxins (chemicals, preservatives, trans fats...) that over time accumulate in the body and congest the organs. As a result, the liver stops burning fat, the pancreas becomes sluggish and can't break down sugars, the thyroid which regulates metabolism becomes underactive...and you can't lose weight.

2. Detox Your Diet (& Cleanse Elimination Organs: If you hold on to waste, you will see it on your waist. It's that simple. I recommend a 21-day detox twice a year. Also avoid Medications when possible. Pharma Drugs inhibit weight loss. Some even cause weight gain. Drugs are processed by the liver as a poison. And when the liver gets congested and full of toxins, it can no longer burn fat properly, and gallbladder stones start to form.

3. Healthy Digestion: Follow the "10 ways to improve your digestion" on page 47 of this book. Undigested food will turn into waste in your colon and not be eliminated properly. As a result, these toxins will be recycled through your body and make your organs sick. Sick organs no longer function properly which will both cause weight gain and inhibit weight loss. Digestion and Elimination are critical for weight loss.

4. Proper Food Combining: This will take your weight loss to the next level! When you combine food groups properly, you maximize digestion, which in turn helps you lose those extra pounds. (view chart page 106)

5. Make Veggies Your Main Course: The Standard American Diet is a plate with meat and starch as the main course, and veggies on the side. Turn that math around and you'll be MUCH healthier, happier, and lose unwanted weight.

6. Intermittent Fasting: Fasting between meals and allowing a full 12-14 hours between dinner and breakfast helps your body fully digest your food, balance blood sugar, and burn fat faster.

7. Take Probiotics: Not enough healthy bacteria in the intestines will inhibit weight loss. Antibiotics, sugar, junk food, & drugs destroy healthy bacteria in the intestines. Probiotics can help restore the healthy balance of the bacteria in your intestines. However, if you have candida/yeast overgrowth, you will likely need more than just probiotics. Yeast overgrowth will greatly inhibit weight loss.

8. Exercise: This is a no brainer, but I do have to list it because surprisingly, some people think they can lose weight without it. You might lose some weight if you just change your diet. However, you will not be in health, and you will plateau at some point and run into a problem.

9. Sleep: You burn fat and heal in your sleep. Don't skip this step it's crucial for both health and weight loss.

10. Balance Hormones: This is huge for weight loss. The key to balancing hormones at ANY age, especially menopause, is to support your adrenal glands.

Super Foods That Heal

Super foods are foods that contain an unusually high concentration of nutrients.

They are foods that feed and nourish the body at a cellular level to promote health and healing. They build the body up making it strong against disease.

Chia Seeds

- Higher than any other omega 3 source.
- Complete protein.
- High in fiber - good for colon health & balancing blood sugar levels.
- Contain boron, which is essential for bone health.
- Have 2 times more potassium than banana.
- Have 3 times more antioxidants than blueberries.
- Rich in calcium, about 2oz of chia seeds contains 600mg of Calcium, as compared to 120 mg for a cup of milk.

Nutritional Yeast Flakes

- Rich source of bio-available vegetarian protein
- High in B vitamin complex, supporting adrenal function and increasing energy
- Supports immune system
- Helps support ideal intestinal ecology
- Supports liver function
- Supports healthy blood lipids
- Supports healthy blood sugar

RAW unpasteurized Apple Cider Vinegar

- Alkalizes the body helping remove toxins

- Removes lactic acid after working out

- Reduces/cures heartburn

- Fights allergies and clears sinus & throat congestion

- Strengthens immune system

- Boosts metabolism

- Alleviates symptoms of arthritis and gout

- Softens gall bladder stones

- Fights Candida (yeast overgrowth)

- Prevents bladder stones and urinary tract infections

- Kills bacteria and soothes sore throat

- Boosts Energy with vital minerals-potassium, calcium, magnesium, phosphorus, chlorine, sodium, copper, Iron...and live enzymes

- Improves digestion-drink water with 1 tablespoon ACV 30 minutes before a meal

Garlic

- Anti-viral, Anti-bacterial, Anti-fungal

- Anti-microbial

- Improves Immune Function

- Acts as natural antibiotic

- Reduces blood sugar

- Lowers cholesterol

- Kills infections: ear, sinus, Candida.

Coconut Oil

- Causes Weight Loss

- Prevents Heart Diseases

- Healing for Pancreatitis

- Healing to Digestion

- Improves Immune system

- Fights Infection

- Detoxifies Liver

- Prevents Diabetes

- Improves Bone Health

*Because coconut water has the same electrolyte balance as blood (it's "isotonic"), it has been called "the fluid of life." During World War II, it was used as a substitute for intravenous plasma. UC Berkeley Wellness Letter, December 2007

*Coconut water comes from young green/white coconuts

Tibetan Goji Berries

Goji berries have become a popular berry in the past few years. However, there is some confusion with goji berries and wolfberries. They are not the same berry, but marketers have started labeling wolfberries as goji berries. Wolfberries are grown in highly polluted areas of China, and have a different nutrient profile. If you want the real goji berry, look for "Tibetan" goji berries. Goji berries are a true superfood, and have been found to have the following health benefits:

- Cancer prevention
- Heart disease prevention
- Lowering cholesterol
- Improving eye health
- Slowing the aging process
- Stress relief
- Better sleep
- Improve immune system
- Great for skin health
- High in essential fatty acids, amino acids, vitamin A, & Vitamin C
- Anti-inflammatory

Hemp Seeds

- Superior source of protein: contain more required amino acid proteins than milk, meat, or eggs.
- Contains Omega's 3, 6, and 9.
- Contain a wide variety of vitamins and minerals.
- Good for relieving constipation

Cayenne Pepper

- Increases blood circulation (critical for healing)
- Strengthens heart, arteries, capillaries, & nerves
- Prevents migraines
- Digestive aide & cleanses colon
- Eliminates sinus congestion
- Anti-fungal, anti-bacterial
- Anti-Inflammatory
- Causes cancer cells to commit suicide
- Anti-flu & cold
- Rids body of LDL cholesterol (bad cholesterol)

Turmeric

- Natural antiseptic and antibacterial
- Natural liver detoxifier; increases bile flow
- Shown to prevent the spread of cancer
- Anti-inflammatory
- Digestive aide
- Natural pain killer
- Can aide in fat metabolism

Alfalfa

- Alfalfa contains <u>virtually all known vitamins</u> including A, D, E, K, B1,B2,B3,B5, B6, and U (good for peptic ulcers). One of the most mineral rich foods known

- It contains Calcium, Iron, Manganese, Potassium, Phosphorus, Sodium, and Magnesium.

- Contains 8 essential enzymes, and is an effective barrier against bacteria invasion.

- It is also good for kidneys and colon health, and is high in protein.

Marine Phytoplankton

- Contains iodine, which is critical for nourishing the thyroid

- Aids in brain development

- Increases metabolism

- Supports liver and heart health

- Alkalizing and detoxifying

- Contains every nutrient necessary for life

- Exceedingly high in oxygen (disease cannot live in an alkaline oxygenated environment)

Aloe Vera Juice

- Inhibits growth of cancer tumors

- Lowers cholesterol

- Repairs "sludge blood" and reverses "sticky blood"

- Eases inflammation and reduces arthritis pain

- Protects kidneys from kidney disease

- Alkalizes the body, helping to balance overly acidic dietary habits

- Heals ulcers, IBS, Crohn's, and other digestive disorders.

- Reduces high blood pressure naturally

- Nourishes the body with vitamins and minerals

- Accelerates healing from physical burns and radiation burns

- Halts colon cancer

- Heals the intestines and lubricates the digestive tract

- Relieves constipation

- Stabilizes blood sugar and reduces triglycerides in diabetics

- Protects the kidneys from disease

Essential Nutrients

Vitamin A

Alfalfa	Goji Berries
Asparagus	Kale
Broccoli	Kelp
Cantaloupe	Parsley
Carrots	Red Peppers
Collard Greens	Spinach
Dandelion Greens	Spirulina
Egg Yolks	Sweet Potatoes

Vitamin B1 (Thiamine)

Alfalfa	Green Peas
Asparagus	Kelp
Beans	Nutritional Yeast
Broccoli	Nuts
Brussels Sprouts	Oats
Brown Rice	Spirulina
Egg Yolks	Sunflower Seeds

Vitamin B2 (Riboflavin)

Alfalfa	Goats Milk
Beans	Whole Grains
Egg Yolks	Green Peas
Fish	Spinach

Vitamin B3 (Niacin)

Alfalfa	Eggs
Broccoli	Fish
Carrots	Green Peas
Dandelion Greens	Nutritional Yeast
Dates	Nuts

Vitamin B5 (Pantothenic Acid)

Asparagus	Eggs
Avocado	Nutritional Yeast
Beans	Sunflower Seeds
Broccoli	Sweet Potato

Vitamin B6 (Pyridoxin)

All Foods	Eggs
Avocados	Fish
Bananas	Nutritional Yeast
Beans	Sunflower Seeds
Brown Rice	Turkey
Brussels Sprouts	Walnuts
Chicken	Whole Grains

Vitamin B9 (Folic Acid)

Asparagus	Kidney Beans
Barley	Legumes
Black Beans	Mung Beans
Brown Rice	Nutritional Yeast
Chicken	Spinach
Green Leafy Vegetables	Whole Grains

Vitamin B12

Eggs	Nutritional Yeast
Meat	Seafood

Biotin

Egg Yolk	Nutritional Yeast
Meat	Whole Grains

Inositol

Beans	Nutritional Yeast Flakes
Fruits	Vegetables
Lecithin	Whole Grains
Meats	

Vitamin C

Alfalfa	Kale
Avocados	Kelp
Beet Greens	Lemons
Brussels Sprouts	Oranges (fresh)
Broccoli	Papaya
Cantaloupe	Parsley
Citrus Fruits	Pineapple
Dandelion Greens	Rose Hips
Goji Berries	Sweet Peppers
Green Vegetables	Strawberries

Vitamin D

Alfalfa	Eggs
Butter	Salmon
Dandelion Greens	Sweet Potatoes

Vitamin E

Alfalfa	Green Leafy Vegetables
Avocado	Kelp
Beans	Nuts & Seeds
Brown Rice	Olive Oil
Dandelion Greens	Sweet Potatoes
Eggs	Whole Grains

Vitamin K

Alfalfa	Green Leafy Vegetables
Asparagus	Eggs
Broccoli	Kelp
Brussels Sprouts	Oats

Calcium

Alfalfa	Dandelion Greens
Almonds	Green Leafy Vegetables
Asparagus	Kelp
Broccoli	Nutritional Yeast
Chia Seeds	Sesame Seeds

*About 2oz of chia seeds contains 600mg of Calcium, as compared to 120 mg for a cup of milk.

Chromium

Broccoli	Fish
Brown Rice	Nutritional Yeast
Chicken	Turkey
Eggs	Whole Grains

Iodine

Asparagus	Lima Beans
Dulse	Sea Food
Kelp	

(Peanuts block iodine absorption)

Iron

Eggs

Green Leafy Vegetables

Meat

Nutritional Yeast

Sesame Seeds (Tahini)

Whole Grains

Magnesium

Alfalfa

Almonds

Apples

Apricots

Avocados

Bananas

Black Beans

Brown Rice

Dandelion

Green Leafy Vegetables

Kelp

Parsley

Pumpkin Seeds

Quinoa

Sesame Seeds

Sunflower Seed

Potassium

Apple Cider Vinegar (Raw)

Avocados

Beans

Beet Greens

Bananas (& other fruit)

Chia Seeds

Fish

Green Leafy Vegetables

Meat

Nutritional Yeast

Sweet Potatoes

Whole Grains

Zinc

Alfalfa, Dandelion, Eggs, Fish, Kelp, Legumes,
Nutritional Yeast, Parsley, Pumpkin Seeds, Sunflower seeds

Supplements to Avoid

Man cannot recreate the apple, but he certainly tries to...

Vitamins - *groups of chemically related compounds, extracted nutrients that science has tried to reproduce.*

Synthetic Vitamins

- Are not food: They are made in a laboratory, chemically produced, not from food.

- Can be harmful and create deficiencies.

- Can be derived from tar. Ex) Thiamin Mononitrite (B1) is derived from coal tar.

- Very inexpensive to make.

- These are the same vitamins under the name "enriched" on many food labels.

- Isolated- Vitamin C needs *other* vitamins to function properly. By itself it is isolated. (Hence multi-vitamins) But think of a car you put gas in, but not oil. Will it run properly? Or an orchestra where the French Horn is blasting; the body needs harmony. Look at a vitamin label vs. the co-factors in an apple.

- An article "The case against vitamins" published in the Wall Street Journal lists studies that show that vitamins may not be beneficial and can actually cause harm to our bodies. They bring us out of nature's balance.

- Reported on April 14, 1994 in The New England Journal of Medicine was a study in which 29,000 male smokers were given synthetic beta-carotene and synthetic Vitamin E to evaluate the cancer-protective effect of these "vitamins". After 10 years, the men taking the synthetic beta-carotene had an 18% higher rate of lung cancer, more heart attacks, and an 8% higher overall death rate. Those taking synthetic vitamin E had more strokes.

On November 23, 1995, the following was reported in The New England Journal of Medicine: 22,748 pregnant women were given synthetic vitamin A. After four years the study was halted because of a 240% increase in birth defects in babies of women taking 10,000 IU daily, and a 400% increase in birth defects in babies of women taking 20,000 IU a day.

- Reported in Reuters Health, March 3, 2000 was a study on men who took 500 mg of synthetic Vitamin C daily. It was found that over an 18-month period, these men had a 250% increase in the intimamedia lining (inner lining) of the carotid artery. This thickening is an accurate measurement for the progression of atherosclerosis. That is, synthetic Vitamin C induced atherosclerosis, even at a 500 mg dose.

In this chart, I have examples of common vitamins you can find in the synthetic pill form, vs. vitamins in their natural food form. The body does not need chemicals, it needs food.

Vitamin	Synthetic Form of Vitamin	Food Based
A & D	Acetate, Retinal Palmitate, Beta Carotene	Alfalfa, Eggs..
B12	Cyanocobalamin	Nutritional Yeast
B3	Niacin	Broccoli, Carrots
C	Ascorbic Acid	Red Peppers
E	d-Alpha Tocopherol	Green Leafy Vegetables

** "We are not vitamin deficient, we are nutrient deficient" Delia Garcia, MD

30 Day Meal Plan

Every day upon rising:
- Clean Water
- Daily Detox Drink

Breakfast: (choose one of the following each day)
- Fresh Fruit
- Breakfast smoothie of choice (pg 76)
- Chia seed banana pudding
- Whole grain gluten free oatmeal

Snack: (choose one - optional)
- Avocado with unrefined sea salt
- Sprouted nuts and seeds mix (1/4 cup)
- Flaxseed Crackers (see grocery pictures)

Lunch: (choose one of the following each day)
- Napa Salad
- Chick pea salad on a bed of spinach
- Salmon stuffed avocado
- Any other recipe from lunch menu on page 73

Snack: (choose one - optional)
- Sliced cucumber chips dipped in fresh guacamole
- Fresh cut veggies dipped in hummus
- Celery sticks with Almond Butter

Dinner: (choose one of the following each day)
- Mexican Cauliflower Rice and Beans
- Vegetarian Chili
- Turkey Burger topped with zucchini & onion saute
- Chicken Stir Fry
- Egg & bacon bit frittata
- Any other recipe from dinner menu on page 74

Breakfast Recipes

Lunch Recipes

Salad Dressing & Dip Recipes

Dinner Recipes

Vegetable Recipes

20 Healthy Snack Ideas!!

It's always best to snack on fresh fruits and veggies

1. Sprouted Nuts and Seeds Mix
2. Avocado slices
3. Chia Kombucha tea
4. Carrots & Celery dipped in hummus
5. Cucumber sliced dipped in guacamole
6. Celery with Almond butter & raisins
7. Hard boiled eggs
8. 85% (or higher) Dark Chocolate Squares
9. Flaxseed Crackers
10. Uncured organic turkey bacon slices
11. Kale Chips
12. Raw Goat Cheddar Cheese Sticks
13. Vegan Protein Shake (Vega Sport)
14. Apple
15. Fresh Vegetable Juice
16. Fresh Cucumbers and Tomato slices
17. Raw Coconut Flakes
18. Raw Hemp Seeds
19. Raw Dehydrated Zucchini Chips
20. Raw Dehydrated Yam Chips

Water

Drinking *clean* water is essential. Please choose from the following options:

Distilled – all impurities are removed. You will want to re-mineralize with unrefined sea salt. (1/4 tsp per quart)

Reverse Osmosis – 99% impurities are removed. You will want to re-mineralize with unrefined sea salt. (1/4 tsp per quart)

Spring Water – only if you are certain it is high quality. Many spring waters are nothing but tap water.

Berkey Water Filter – may be the best option if you're in the market to buy a system.

Avoid *tap water* as much as possible especially during your detox. *Carbon filters* are not a good choice either.

Daily Detox Drink

Water 3-4 ounces, (more is fine). I use a large shot glass and shoot the drink down fast :)

Fresh lemon juice - 1 Tbsp - Cleanses & stimulates digestion, alkalizes & neutralizes harmful acids.

Raw Apple Cider Vinegar - 1 Tbsp - Alkalizing, anti-bacterial, fights candida, & digestive aid.

Oceans - Boosts immune system, high in oxygen, alkalizing minerals, amino acids, enzymes, Omega 3's, detoxifying, nourishing.

See Video for Alternative Tastier Detox Drink Recipe ☺

Fresh Fruit

Ingredients:

Strawberries	Pineapple
Grapes	Apple
Cherries	Grapefruit

Instructions:
Choose **ONE** of the above types of fruit, and eat until full. Allow 1 hour before eating any other food.

Banana Berry Green Smoothie

Ingredients:
10-16oz cold water depending on how thick you like it
2 hands full Leafy Greens (kale, spinach, collards...)
3/4 cup frozen organic berries
1/2 frozen banana (peel before freezing)
Stevia to taste (optional)

Instructions:
Fill blender cup with greens first
Add cold water and blend

Hemp Seed Banana Smoothie

Ingredients:
10oz unsweetened chocolate or vanilla almond milk
1 frozen banana (peel before freezing)
3 tablespoons raw hemp seeds
Stevia to taste (optional)

Instructions:
Blend until smooth and enjoy!

Alternate Version: Add 2 handfuls of spinach

Chia Seed Banana Pudding

Ingredients:

6oz unsweetened almond milk (or purified water)
2 Tbsp organic chia seeds
1 Ripe banana
Stevia to taste (optional)

Instructions:

Add chia seeds to water
Stir frequently until it starts to gel
Refrigerate until you're ready to use it
Next morning - add sliced banana pieces to the chia gel, stir and enjoy

Gluten Free Whole Grain Oats

Ingredients:

Gluten Free Whole Grain Oats (no sugar or preservatives)
Water (amount per instructions on container)
1 teaspoon coconut oil or ghee
Stevia to taste
Cinnamon to taste

Instructions:

Prepare according to instruction on the bag & add stevia, cinnamon, and coconut oil or ghee

Black Bean Salad

Ingredients:
1 large can black beans
1 tbsp Olive Oil
2 tbsp raw apple cider vinegar
Sea salt to taste
1/4 sweet onion chopped
1 red pepper chopped
1 carrot chopped

Instructions:
Mix all ingredients in a large bowl, refrigerate, and serve

**Alternate Version: *Substitue veggies with cherry tomatoes and avocado.*

Black Bean Quinoa Salad

Ingredients:
1 cup uncooked quinoa, rinsed
1/4 onion chopped
1 red bell pepper chopped
1 15 ounce can black beans, rinsed and drained
1 tbsp olive oil
2 tbsp raw apple cider vinegar (ACV)
1/2 tsp salt

Instructions:
Cook quinoa according to package directions. Set aside and let cool. Whisk together olive oil, ACV, salt and pepper. Add red bell pepper and black beans to quinoa. Gently stir in lime juice mixture. For best results, refrigerate for 30 minutes before serving.

Egg Salad Wraps

Ingredients:

3 Eggs (hard boiled)
1 Tbsp onions chopped
1/2 celery stalk chopped
Paleo Mayonaise to taste
Romaine lettus
Sea salt and pepper to taste

Instructions:

Peel hard boiled eggs
Remove yolks and mix with other ingredients
Cut egg whites into small pieces
Add egg whites to mixture
Serve on romaine lettuce leaves

Chick Pea Salad

Ingredients:

1 can chick peas
1 can kidney beans
1/2 cup chopped
scallions
1/2 red pepper chopped
1 carrot chopped

1 zucchini chopped
Olive oil
Spinach
Unrefined sea salt
Raw apple cider vinegar
(or lemon juice)

Salad Dressing:

2 tablespoons RAW apple cider vinegar
1 tablespoons olive oil
2 pressed garlic cloves
Unrefined Sea Salt to taste
If you prefer less oil feel free to modify the salad dressing accordingly.
Also, just a note, unrefined Sea Salt is more salty tasting than refined table salt.

Instructions:

Drain and rinse beans
Pour chick peas and kidney beans into a bowl
Chop up all the veggies and add to the beans
Mix Salad Dressing and stir thoroughly into ingredients
Refrigerate and serve cold on a bed of spinach

**Alternate version: Substitute veggies with cucumber, cherry tomatoes, and add Paleo Mayonaise (in place of salad dressing)*

Mason Jar Lunch

Ingredients:

1 (19-oz.) can chickpeas, drained and rinsed
1 tablespoon chopped fresh flat-leaf parsley
1 tablespoon chopped fresh mint
1 tablespoon fresh lemon juice
2 tablespoons olive oil
3/4 cup chopped radishes
1/8 cup finely chopped red onion
1 pt. grape tomatoes, halved
1 1/2 cups chopped English cucumbers
Lemon wedges

Instructions:

Stir together first 4 ingredients and 1 Tbsp. olive oil; Add unrefined salt and black pepper to taste; let stand 15 minutes.

Meanwhile, stir together radishes, onion, tomatoes and cucumbers with remaining olive oil. Season with salt and pepper to taste.

In a mason jar : Layer ½ chickpea mixture, then ½ radish, tomato and cucumber mixture. Repeat . Cover and chill 2 to 4 hours. Serve with lemon wedges and *Mary's Gone Crackers*

**Alternate Version: *Replace chick peas with 2 cooked boneless skinless chicken breasts chopped.*

Recipe by Margie Setterlof, MS

Napa Salad

Ingredients:
4 cups Napa cabbage
1 carrot chopped or sliced
1/2 cucumber chopped
1/2 red pepper chopped
1/2 avocado cut into peices

Salad Dressing:
Fresh squeezed lemon juice with a drizzle of olive oil

Instructions: Mix all ingredients in a salad bowl, mash the avocado, and add dressing.

Romaine Spinach Salad

Ingredients:
4 cups Romaine Lettuce
1 cup spinach
1 carrot sliced
1 radishe sliced
1/2 red bell pepper chopped
1 Tablespoon raw sprouted sunflower seeds
1/2 avocado cut into pieces

Instructions:
Mix all ingredients in a salad bowl, add Miso salad dressing (or homemade Mediterranean Salad Dressing if you are on the elimination diet), and serve.

Salmon Salad Lettuce Wraps

Ingredients:

1 small can or pouch of wild caught salmon
1 tablespoon *Paleo* Mayonnaise
1/4 cup chopped celery
1 teaspoon lime
Unrefined sea salt & pepper to taste
Romaine lettuce

Instructions:

Mix salmon with *Paleo Mayonaise*
Add celery, lime, and seasonings
Wrap in romaine leaf and serve

Salmon Tossed Salad

Ingredients:

2 cups cooked, flaked salmon (bake or broil), or wild caught canned
1 red or green bell pepper, diced
1 cucumber, peeled, seeded, and diced
½ cup chopped onions
½ cup chopped scallions
4-5 tbsp *Paleo mayonaise* or enough to moisten
¼ tsp cayenne pepper
salt and pepper
salad ready romaine lettuce for base
½ lemon, juiced

Instructions:

Place salmon in large bowl. In another bowl, combine bell pepper, cucumber, onion, and vegan mayo. Add seasonings and stir to combine. Pour mixture over salmon, add lemon juice and toss lightly to combine. Serve over romaine lettuce.

Recipe by Margie Setterlof, MS

Black Bean Salsa

Ingredients:
2 cans of black beans (drained)
1 & 1/2 cups frozen or fresh organic corn
1/2 cup Grapeseed Vegenaise Mayo
1 lime juiced
1/2 cup chopped red onion
12 cherry tomatoes halved
1/4 cup cilantro chopped
Unrefined sea salt and pepper to taste

Instructions:
Mix lime juice and mayo in large bowl
Add cilantro and onion and mix
Add the rest of the ingredients
Add sea salt and pepper to taste
Mix and refrigerate

Mung Bean Salad

Ingredients:
1 cup dry mung beans
1 carrot shredded
2 tablespoons scallions chopped
1/2 celery stalk
2 tablespoons fresh squeezed lemon juice
1 tablespoon olive oil
Unrefined Sea Salt to taste

Instructions:
Soak mung beans in 2 cups purified water overnight
Put just the mung beans in a sauce pan with new water about 1/2 inch above the beans
Bring to a boil, then simmer about 20 minutes until soft, but not mushy.
Drain remaining water
Add carrot, scallions, celery, lemon juice & olive oil
Unrefined sea salt to taste
Refrigerate and serve cold

Salmon Stuffed Avocados

Ingredients:

1 avocado, halved and pitted
1 small can wild caught salmon
1/2 chopped red bell pepper
1 Tbsp chopped onion
1 tablespoon lemon juice
salt and pepper to taste

Instructions:

1 avocado, halved and pitted
1 small can wild caught salmon
1/2 chopped red bell pepper
1 Tbsp chopped onion
1 tablespoon lemon juice
salt and pepper to taste

Zoodle Salad

Ingredients:

Supplies: _Veggetti Spiral Vegetable Maker_ (or grate)
Spinach or Romaine lettuce
1 carrot (spiral using _Veggetti)_
1/2 green zucchini squash (spiral using _Veggetti_)
4-5 sliced grape tomatos
Onion slices to taste
Salad dressing of choice (page 94)

Instructions:

Combine ingredients in a large bowl
Add homeade salad dressing and serve
(Purchase "Veggetti" on line or Bed Bath and Beyond)

Chicken & Cauliflower Rice

Ingredients:
1-2 chicken breasts (or thighs)
Cooked cauliflower rice (see recipe page 93)
1 tablespoon of ghee

Instructions:
Preheat oven to 350 degrees
Place chicken in baking dish
Bake 40 minutes
While baking chicken - cook cauliflower rice
Fill plate with cooked cauliflower rice
Place baked chicken on cauliflower rice and serve

Wild Caught Salmon & Veggies

Ingredients:
8 ounce piece of Halibut, <u>Wild Caught</u> Salmon
2 carrots (or another veggy of choice)
1 tablespoon ghee melted
Fresh sqeezed lemon juice
Mrs. Dash (or fresh herbs)

Instructions:
Preheat oven to 400 degrees
Place fish in baking dish
Add carrots to baking dish
Add water to cover the bottom of the dish
Drizzle fish and carrots with ghee (or dip in small dish of melted ghee)
Mrs Dash to taste
Bake for 35-40 minutes and serve

Eggs & Bacon Bit Frittata

Ingredients:
8 eggs, whisked
2 slices uncured turkey bacon (fried)
1/4 onion chopped
2 garlic cloves
Large handful of spinach
1 tablespoon Ghee
Unrefined sea salt
Pepper

Instructions:
Saute onion, garlic, spinach in ghee 5-7 minutes
Add to baking dish with eggs
Add sea salt and pepper to taste
Bake for 20 minutes at 375 degrees F

Goat Feta Chicken Bake

Ingredients:
6 boneless skinless chicken breasts (1-1/2 lb.)
2 Tbsp. lemon juice, divided
¼ tsp. black pepper
4 oz. Crumbled **GOAT** Feta Cheese (technically dairy)
¼ cup finely chopped red peppers
¼ cup finely chopped fresh parsley
Fresh basil

Instructions:
Heat oven to 350°F.
Place chicken in 13x9-inch baking dish (coat pan with ghee or coconut oil)
Drizzle with 1 Tbsp. lemon juice. Season with black pepper. Top with feta cheese; drizzle with remaining lemon juice.
Bake 35 to 40 min. or until chicken is done (165°F). Top with red peppers, fresh parsley and basil

Recipe by Margie Setterlof, MS

Chicken Vegetable Soup

Ingredients:
One pound of boneless chicken thighs (or breast meat)
2-3 teaspoon unrefined sea salt
2-3 teaspoon Mrs. Dash Table Blend
4 garlic cloves
4 carrots
1 bunch asparagus
4 celery stalks chopped
1 onion or leek chopped
1 turnip chopped (or skin of 4 potatoes-1/8th inch thick)

Instructions:
Place chicken in crock pot
Add sea salt, Mrs. Dash, and ghee
Add veggies
Add enough purified water to cover all veggies (should be about 8-10 cups)
Cook in crock pot on high for 4 hours
Ready to serve

Rice Congee (Rice Soup)

Ingredients:
9 cups water (use less water for thinner soup)

2 cups brown rice	1 onion chopped
2 minced garlic cloves	4 celery sticks chopped
2-3 teaspoons sea salt	4 carrot sticks chopped
4 chicken thighs	1 tablespoon Ghee

Instructions:
Place all of the ingredients in a 3-quart soup pot. Bring to a boil, lower the heat to very slow simmer and cook for at least 1.5 hours. (Or, place in a crock pot and cook on high for about 5 hours.) Add additional water if needed.

Not proper food combining but easy to digest

Spaghetti Squash & Fire Roasted Tomatos

Ingredients:
1 whole spaghetti squash
1 can fire roasted tomatos
2-3 garlic cloves
1/4 cup onion chopped
1 cup fresh asaparagus chopped
1 tablespoon ghee or coconut oil

Instructions:
Place whole (uncut) spaghetti squash on a parchment paper lined baking sheet
Bake at 350° for 60-80 minutes
Allow spaghetti squash to cool for 20-30 minutes
Cut squash open with a knife
Using a spoon scoop out seeds
Scrape the flesh out of the squash into stringy noodles and place on large plate

In Skillet
Sautee garlic, onion, and asparagus in ghee
Add fire roasted tomatoes, cook on medium low until hot
Add to plate of spaghetti squash and serve

Vegetarian Chili

Step 1:

In large pot sweat (saute) the following:
2 tablespoons Ghee
1/2 large onion chopped
4-6 garlic cloves
1 teaspoon fresh ginger chopped finely
Jalapenos to taste (optional)
1 1/2 teaspoon unrefined sea salt
Pepper to taste

Step 2:
Add the following veggies to the large pot:
16oz Imagine Chicken Broth
1 can each of kidney beans, pinto beans, black beans
2 small zucchini chopped
1 pound fresh asparagus chopped (I only use top halves)
2 carrots chopped
1 cup frozen corn
2 cans diced tomatoes
3 teaspoons chili powder
Simmer 30-45 minutes and serve

Kale Quinoa

Ingredients:
2/3 cup cooked Quinoa (instructions are on the bag)
1 bunch of chopped kale (baby kale works well)
1 Garlic Clove
1 Tbsp ghee
Unrefined sea salt

Instructions:
Bring 2/3 cup water and quinoa to a boil in a saucepan.
Reduce heat to medium-low, cover, and simmer until
quinoa is tender and water has been absorbed, 15-20
minutes
Heat ghee in a skillet, saute garlic and kale until kale is
wilted
Stir quinoa into kale mixture, salt, and serve

Sweet Potato & Veggies

Ingredients:
1 sweet potato (cut into bite sized pieces)
Steamed Broccoli (or other veggie)
1 tablespoon of ghee
Unrefined sea salt

Instructions:
Preheat oven to 350 degrees
Place sweet potato in baking dish
Add water to cover the bottom of the dish
Melt ghee and drizzle on sweet potato
Unrefined sea salt to taste
Bake for 45-50 minutes
Steam brocoli in separate pan
Drizzle ghee over broccoli
Serve with sweet potato

Turkey Burgers

Ingredients:
1 pound organic ground turkey (thigh works best)
1 teaspoon Redmonds Real Salt
1/4 onion finely chopped

Instructions:
Mix ingredients in a bowl
Form into patties and grill
Serve on bed of romaine

**Alternate Version: *Turn your turkey burger meal into a healthy casserole. Break up your burger into smaller pieces, and pour sauteed zuchini & onions on top of chopped up burger.*

Mexican Cauliflower Rice & Beans

Ingredients:
1 tablespoon ghee
2 cups cauliflower rice (grated cauliflower)
1/2 cup cooked pinto beans
1/4 cup fresh cilantro
1/2 fresh lime squeezed
garlic powder
onion powder
chili powder
cumin powder
paprika powder
sea salt
pepper

Instructions:
In a pan, melt ghee over medium high heat
Cook garlic, cauliflower rice, pinto beans 5-10 minutes
Add a few shakes of each seasoning listed, mix and serve

Chicken Stir Fry

Ingredients:
2 boneless Chicken Thighs (or chicken breast)
1 bag organic frozen stir fry veggies
OR all fresh veggies (carrot, celery, chopped onion, broccoli and red pepper)
"Coconut Secret" Coconut Aminos (Soy Sauce)

Instructions:
Cut chicken into small pieces, place in skillet
Add coconut aminos, simmer med low until cooked
Add veggies (fresh or frozen)
Turn heat up to medium high
Stir often until veggies are cooked yet slightly crunchy

Taco Lettuce Wraps

Ingredients:
1 lbs ground turkey (thigh meat)
1 tsp garlic powder
1 tsp cumin
1 tsp salt
1 tsp chili powder
1 tsp paprika
1/2 small onion, minced
4 oz can tomato sauce
3 Romaine lettuce leaves
Shredded goat cheese

Instructions
Brown turkey in a large skillet with onion
Let turkey cool, break up finely
Turn back to medium low
Add dry seasoning and tomato sauces
Simmer on low for about 10 minutes
Place mixture on romaine lettuce leafs
Top with shredded goat cheese and serve!

Garlic Asparagus

Ingredients:
1 pound fresh asparagus cut into small pieces
1 tablespoon ghee
1 garlic clove finely chopped
Unrefined sea salt

Instructions:
Melt ghee in large skillet on low heat
Add asparagus and garlic
Cook until you can put a fork in it
Add sea salt, and serve

Cooked Kale

Ingredients:
4 cups raw kale (cut up)
1 tablespoon coconut oil
1/4 cup sweet onion chopped
1 garlic clove crushed

Instructions:
Melt coconut in large skillet on low heat

Add onion, garlic, and kale
Simmer, stir often, until kale wilts
Ready to serve

Cilantro Lime Cauliflower Rice

Ingredients:
1 tablespoon ghee
2 cups cauliflower rice (grated cauliflower)
1 garlic clove minced
1 tsp fresh squeezed lime juice (half a lime)
2 Tbsp fresh cilantro (or 1 tsp dried cilantro)
Unrefined sea salt and pepper to taste

Instructions:
In a pan, melt ghee over medium high heat
Cook garlic, cauliflower, 5-10 minutes
Mix in cilantro
Add sea salt, pepper, and lime to taste and serve

Fresh Green Beans & Onions

Ingredients:
2-4 cups fresh green beans
1/4 thinly sliced onion
1 tablespoon ghee
Redmonds Real Salt or Mrs. Dash

Instructions:
Pour enough purified water in a skillet to cover the bottom thoroughly
Turn the stove on to a med low heat
Add green beans & onion (stir often)
Steam 5-7 minutes, until zucchini & onion slices are still slightly crunchy
Drizzle melted ghee on top
Ready to serve

Mashed Parsnips

Ingredients:
1 parsnip
2 tablespoons of ghee
Unrefined sea salt and pepper to taste

Instructions:
Cut turnip into 1/2" size peices
Place in a pan and cover with water
Boil until turnips are fork soft
Drain water and mash
Add ghee, seasonings, and enjoy

**Alternate Version: Replace parsnips in place of turnips.

Zucchini Zoodles

Ingredients:
1 spiralize zucchini with a spiralizer
1/4 thinly sliced onion
1 tablespoon ghee
Redmonds Real Salt or Mrs. Dash

Instructions:
Pour thin layer of water in pan
Turn the stove on to a med low heat
Add ghee and melt
Add zucchini & onion (stir often)
Cook 5-7 minutes and serve

Raw Mixed Veggies

Ingredients:
1 cup cabbage chopped
2-4 radishes grated
1 carrot grated
1 red pepper chopped
1 cup jicama chopped
1 celery stick chopped

Instructions:
Chop veggies
Add a home made salad dressing from salad dressing recipe's
Ready to serve

Stuffed Portobello Mushrooms

Ingredients:
2 Portobello Mushrooms
1/2 Cup chopped onion
2 Garlic cloves
3 Handfuls of spinach
1/2 Can fire roasted tomatoes
MCT oil (or melted ghee)
Sea Salt

Instructions:
Preheat oven to 375 degrees F
Rinse mushrooms
Cut stem out of mushrooms
Brush both sides of mushrooms with MCT oil (or melted ghee)
Place in a baking dish inside up

In a skillet:
Chop and saute the following for 7-10 minutes on medium low in MCT oil
Onion
Garlic
Spinach
Fire roasted tomatoes
Salt to taste

Last Step:
Fill mushrooms with sauteed veggies
Bake for 20 minutes
Serve and enjoy!

Salad Dressings

Mediterranean Salad Dressing

Ingredients:
3 tablespoons Extra Virgin Olive Oil
1 tablespoon fresh squeezed lemon juice
1 fresh pressed garlic clove
Unrefined Sea Salt to taste

Instructions:
Press or chop garlic clove into the olive oil & let sit for
5 minutes or more
Add lemon juice, pour into a cruet bottle & mix well

Avocado Salad Dressing

Ingredients:
1/2 avocado
1/2 lemon squeezed fresh
Pinch of dill or basil
Unrefined sea salt to taste

Instructions:
Mash avocado, mix with other ingredients, and pour
over salad

Creamy Ranch Dressing

Ingredients:
1/2 cup *Paleo* Mayonnaise
1/2 tsp. garlic powder (not garlic salt)
1 tsp. minced onion
1 tsp. fresh lemon juice
1/4 tsp. Unrefined Sea salt
1-2 tablespoons purified water (leave out for dip)

Instructions:
Mix well and pour into a dish or cruet bottle.

Pico De Gallo

Ingredients:
2 organic tomatoes diced
1 garlic clove, peeled and diced
1/4 medium sized onion diced
Juice of 1 lime
1-2 Tablespoons cilantro leaves, chopped
1 jalapeno diced (optional)
Unrefined sea salt to taste

Instructions:
Combine ingredients in a bowl and refrigerate for 30 minutes.
Serve with Mary's Gone Crackers or fresh sliced cucumber or zuchini.

Guacamole

Ingredients:
1 Avocado
1/4 cup chopped onion
Fresh lime juice to taste
1/2 ripe tomato
Unrefined sea salt
Cucumber sliced

Instructions:
Cut avocado in half, remove seed and peel, place in mixing bowl. Mash avocado with onion, tomato, lime juice, and sea salt.

Dip cucumber slices into guacamole and enjoy!

**Alternate option: Layer pico de gallo over guacamole

Ghee Recipe

Ingredients:

1 pound organic no salt butter

Instructions:

1. Place all 4 sticks of butter in a pan

2. Turn to med low heat (level 4 if you have an electric stove)

3. After butter melts you will see a white foam on top, skim gently as much as you can.

4. The butter will "boil" and sound like crackling, let cook like this or about 7 minutes. Watch bottom of pan, you will see the milk solids (white) start to stick to the bottom.

5. Keep checking bottom. As soon as you see any brown (burnt milk solids) on bottom, immediately remove from the heat.

6. Strain with cheese cloth into a glass jar and let cool.

7. Store unrefrigerated. Always use a clean dry spoon or knife so it doesn't spoil, and it will last about a year.

Grocery List

*Common allergens for the elimination diet

Fruit

Apples

Apricots

Bananas

Blackberries

Blueberries

Cantaloupe

Cherries

Cranberries

Grapefruit

Grapes

Melon

Kiwi Fruit

Kumquats

Lemons

Limes

Mangoes

Nectarines

Oranges*

Papayas

Passion Fruit

Peaches

Pears

Persimmons

Pineapple

Plantains

Plums

Pomegranates

Raspberries

Strawberries*

Tangerines

Waterm

Food Combining:

Eat fruit by itself in the morning, 2 hours before any other food. Melons are best not mixed with other fruits.

Vegetables

Artichoke	Jicama
Asparagus	Kale
Bamboo Shoots	Leeks
Beets	Romaine lettuce
Beet Greens	Mushrooms
Bell Peppers	Okra
Bok Choy	Onions
Broccoli	Parsnips
Cabbage	Radicchio
Carrots	Radishes
Cauliflower	Rhubarb
Celery	Rutabaga
Cabbage	Scallions
Collard greens	Snow peas
Cucumbers	Spinach
Daikon	Squash
Eggplant	Swiss chard
Fennel	Tomatoes *
Green beans	Turnips
Green Peas	Watercress
Mustard greens	Zucchini

Food Combining: Vegetables can be eaten with any food anytime with the exception of fruit

Protein

Organic antibiotic free chicken or turkey

Eggs*

Hemp Seeds

Wild Caught Fish

Avocados

Raw plant-based protein powder

Sprouted sunflower seeds

Raw walnuts (soak in water 12 hours)

Sprouted pumpkin seeds

Raw Pecans (soak in water 12 hours)

Chia seeds

Organic almond butter or sunflower seed butter

Unsweetened Almond or Coconut Milk

Food Combining:

Animal protein should only be combined with vegetables (and fats if you take digestive enzymes)

Avoid mixing animal proteins with plant proteins. (For example: nuts or seeds do not combine well with chicken breast)

Grains & Starches

Beans

Brown rice

Quinoa

Millet

Buckwheat

Spelt

Amaranth

Sweet Potato

(*Avoid foods in italics if you have yeast overgrowth*)

Food Combing: Carbs/Starches can be eaten with veggies and fats.

Fats

Cold pressed extra virgin coconut oil

Cold pressed extra virgin olive oil

Ghee (made from organic no salt butter)

Food Combining:

Fats can be eaten with starches OR proteins.
Do not combine fats with both starch AND protein

Herbs and Spices

Unrefined Sea Salt

Raw Apple Cider*

Vinegar*

Basil

Bay Leaves

Cilantro

Dill

Marjoram

Mint

Oregano

Parsley

Rosemary

Sage

Tarragon

Thyme

Anise

Coconut Aminos*

Cardamom

Caraway

Cayenne Pepper

Cinnamon

Fennel

Fresh Ground Black

Pepper

Garlic

Ginger

Mustard Powder

Nutmeg

Paprika

Turmeric

Food Combining:

Herbs combine well with any food

Foods That Heal You
Proper Food Combining Chart
To Maximize Digestion & Weight Loss

Only Combine where boxes touch directly

Acid Fruits	Sub Acid Fruits	Sweet Fruits
Lemons, Limes	Apples, Pears	Bananas
Strawberries	Berries	Grapes
Oranges, Grapefruit	Sweet Cherries	Mangos
Pineapples	Plums, Peaches	Papaya
Tomato	Kiwi	Dried Fruit

Starches	Meat	Nuts & Seeds
Grains, Rice, Oats	Beef, Chicken	Almonds, Walnuts
Pasta, Crackers	Turkey, Fish	Coconuts
Bread, Corn, Beans	Dairy, Eggs, Milk	Seeds: Chia
Potatoes	Cheese,...	Flax, Hemp,
Yams, Squash	Protein Powders	Sunflower Seeds

Veggies		
Asparagus	Eggplant	Cucumber, Celery
Beets	Green Beans	Spinach, Kale
Broccoli	Green Peas	Turnips
Brussels	Leeks, Onions	Zucchini (summer)
Cabbage	Dandelion	Cauliflower

Exceptions

Leafy Greens—combine well with ANYTHING even fruit

Melons—do not mix with ANY other food, not even other fruit

Bananas & Dried Fruit: combine well with nuts and seeds

Avocados: combine best with fruit, veggies, or starches

Lemons: combine well with veggies, nuts, seeds (not w/starch or protein)

Oils/Fats: Combine with anything BUT fruit

Healing Prayer

Heavenly Father, I believe (according to Isaiah 53) that you made me whole 2000 years ago on the cross through the blood of Jesus. And I ask in the name of Jesus (according to John 14:14 & Matthew 7:7), that you will help me to trust you; cause me to receive your gift of divine health in my body, soul, and spirit, and cause me to prosper in every area of my life. Come Holy Spirit and release God's favor in my life today, purify me through the blood of Jesus, and fill me with the Father's Healing Light from the top of my head to the soles of my feet. Heavenly Father I also ask that you will have mercy on me and forgive me for holding on to any anger, pain, un-forgiveness, unbelief, sadness, fear, shock or trauma. And I choose right now in Jesus name to let go of all of it, and release it to you at the cross as I receive your love, your peace, your freedom, your grace, your redemption, your forgiveness, and your divine health.
"To the praise of His glorious grace" in Jesus name I pray, Amen.

Nutrition & Health Coaching Services

- One-On-One Nutrition & Health Coaching

- 21 Day Detoxification Program By Catherine Rudolph CNC.,
  To Cleanse Colon, Kidney, Liver, Lung, Lymph, & Skin

- FREE Teaching Video Library

Catherine Rudolph, C.N.C.
Complete Rapha Nutrition, LLC
FoodsThatHealyou@gmail.com
www.FoodsThatHealYou.com
317-698-6150

*A special thanks to Marie Andorfer
for her editing assistance*

18729032R00062

Made in the USA
Middletown, DE
01 December 2018